# MULTIPLE SCLEROSIS ANTI-INFLAMMATORY COOKBOOK

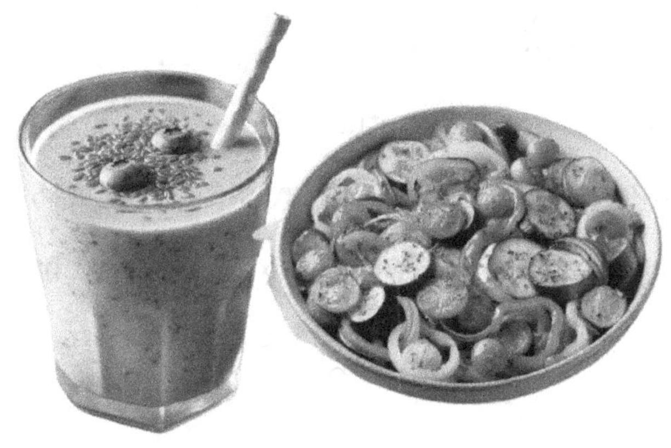

*A Guide to Healthy Eating for People with MS*

## NOREEN HART

# Copyright © 2023 by Noreen Hart

# TABLE OF CONTENTS

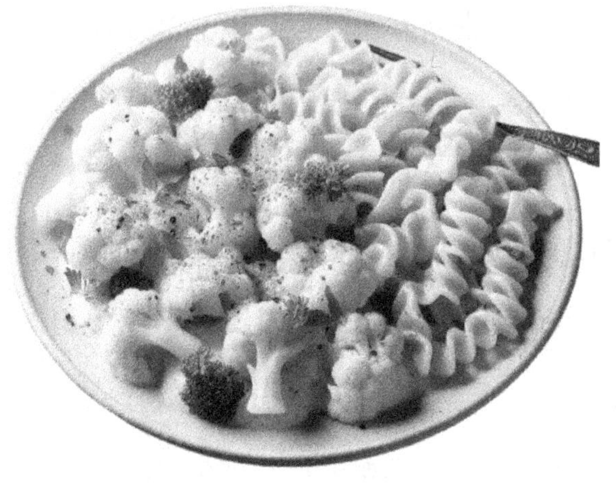

## DISCLAIMER

The information provided in this book is intended for general informational purposes only and should not be considered a substitute for professional medical advice. While we have taken great care to provide accurate and up-to-date information, it is essential to consult with a qualified healthcare professional before making significant dietary changes, especially if you have been diagnosed with multiple sclerosis or any other medical condition.

The recipes in this cookbook have been designed to follow the principles of a multiple sclerosis diet, but individual dietary requirements may vary. We encourage you to consider your health, preferences, and any food allergies or sensitivities when using these recipes.

The authors, publisher and any related parties do not assume responsibility for any adverse effects, allergic reactions, or health issues that may result from using or misusing the recipes or information provided in this cookbook.

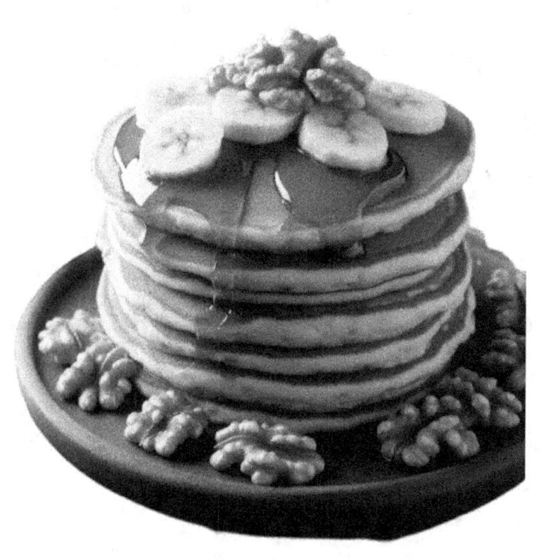

# INTRODUCTION

Welcome to the **"Multiple Sclerosis Anti-Inflammatory Cookbook."** This book is your guide to understanding the profound connection between diet and managing the symptoms of multiple sclerosis (MS).

Whether you have been recently diagnosed with MS or have been living with the condition for some time, this cookbook is designed to empower you with the knowledge and recipes you need to embrace a healthier, more vibrant lifestyle.

Multiple sclerosis, a complex neurological disorder, affects millions of individuals around the globe. While there is no known cure, there are ways to manage the symptoms and improve the quality of life for those living with MS. One of the most promising approaches to managing MS is through dietary choices.

This book is not just a collection of recipes; it is a comprehensive resource that will walk you through the principles of the MS diet, the benefits it can offer, and a practical guide to incorporating it into your daily life. I believe that what you eat can have a profound impact on your health, energy levels, and overall well-being.

In the following pages, you will find a carefully curated selection of delicious and nutritious recipes that align with the principles of the MS diet. These recipes are not only designed to be healthy but also enjoyable, ensuring that your journey toward wellness is not only sustainable but also satisfying.

As you explore the pages of this cookbook, you'll discover an array of breakfasts, lunches, dinners, snacks, and beverages, each thoughtfully created to meet your nutritional needs and tantalize your taste buds. Additionally, you'll find a 30-day meal plan to help you get started on your MS diet journey.

I invite you to embark on this culinary adventure with me, so we can explore how food can be a powerful tool in managing multiple sclerosis. Together, we'll discover that with the right ingredients and a mindful approach to nutrition, you can take control of your health and savor the flavors of a life well-lived, even in the face of challenges.

Let's begin this transformative journey towards a healthier and happier you through the **"Multiple Sclerosis Anti-Inflammatory Cookbook."**

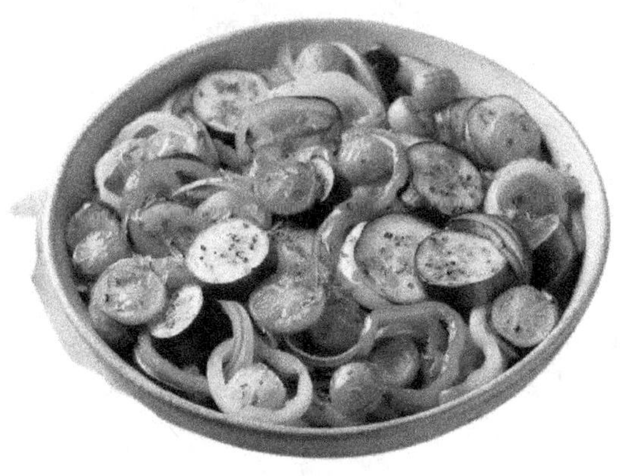

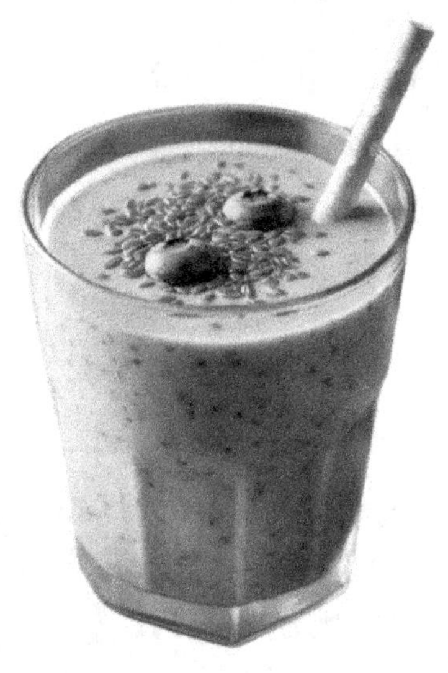

# CHAPTER 1

## Principles of the multiple sclerosis diet

Managing multiple sclerosis through diet is about making informed choices to support your overall well-being. These are the essential principles to bear in mind:

1. **Balanced Nutrition:** The MS diet emphasizes a balance of macronutrients—proteins, carbohydrates, and healthy fats—to provide essential energy and promote overall health.

2. **Anti-Inflammatory Foods:** Incorporate foods rich in antioxidants, like colorful fruits and vegetables, which can help reduce inflammation in the body.

3. **Omega-3 Fatty Acids:** Consume sources of omega-3 fatty acids, such as fatty fish,

flaxseeds, and walnuts, to support brain health and reduce inflammation.

4. **Whole Grains:** Choose whole grains over refined ones for sustained energy and fiber, helping with digestion and maintaining stable blood sugar levels.

5. **Lean Proteins:** Opt for lean protein sources like poultry, beans, and tofu to support muscle strength and repair.

6. **Vitamin D:** Adequate vitamin D intake is vital for those with MS, as it plays a role in immune function. Consider supplements, as sunlight exposure may be limited.

7. **Hydration:** Staying well-hydrated is essential. Water and herbal teas can help with symptom management.

8. **Portion Control:** Be mindful of portion sizes to maintain a healthy weight and prevent overeating, which can lead to fatigue.

9. **Limit Processed Foods:** Minimize processed and high-sugar foods that can contribute to inflammation and energy fluctuations.

10. **Personalization:** While these are general principles, it's crucial to personalize your diet to your specific needs and consult with a healthcare provider or nutritionist if necessary.

These principles serve as a foundation for the recipes and meal plans you'll find in this cookbook. By adhering to these guidelines, you can make more conscious and health-conscious choices, potentially helping to manage your multiple sclerosis symptoms and enhance your quality of life.

## Benefits of Multiple Sclerosis Diet

Adopting a well-considered diet tailored to the needs of multiple sclerosis can bring about various advantages for those managing this condition:

1. **Reduced Inflammation:** The MS diet is designed to contain anti-inflammatory foods,

which can help decrease the overall inflammation in the body. This reduction in inflammation may alleviate MS symptoms and enhance comfort.

2. **Enhanced Energy Levels:** A diet focused on nutrient-rich, whole foods can contribute to increased energy levels, helping to counteract the fatigue commonly associated with MS.

3. **Improved Digestion:** The emphasis on high-fiber foods in the diet can promote better digestion and help mitigate digestive issues that individuals with MS may experience.

4. **Better Immune Support:** Specific nutrients and antioxidants in the diet can support the immune system, possibly helping to reduce the risk of relapses.

5. **Weight Management:** Adopting a diet that encourages portion control and limits processed foods can contribute to maintaining

a healthy weight, which is vital for those with MS.

6. **Enhanced Mental Well-Being:** The nutritional benefits of the diet may lead to improved mental clarity, memory, and overall cognitive function, supporting emotional well-being.

7. **Optimized Muscle Function:** The inclusion of lean proteins in the diet can promote muscle strength and function, crucial for maintaining mobility and overall health.

8. **Disease Progression Control:** Although diet alone cannot cure MS, it can potentially help manage symptoms and slow disease progression.

By embracing the principles of the MS diet and incorporating the recipes in this cookbook, you are taking significant steps toward nurturing your overall health and well-being. While the benefits may vary from person to person, the potential improvements in quality of life make this dietary approach a valuable consideration for those living with multiple sclerosis.

## Foods to Eat

The Multiple Sclerosis Diet focuses on incorporating a variety of nutrient-rich foods that can provide essential vitamins, minerals, and support for those managing MS. Here are some key foods to include:

1. **Fruits and Vegetables:** Load up on a colorful array of fruits and vegetables. These are rich in antioxidants and essential vitamins to reduce inflammation and boost overall health.

2. **Fatty Fish:** Salmon, mackerel, and sardines are excellent sources of omega-3 fatty acids, which support brain health and reduce inflammation.

3. **Whole Grains:** Choose whole grains like quinoa, brown rice, and oats for their high fiber content, promoting steady energy levels.

4. **Lean Proteins:** Incorporate lean protein sources such as poultry, beans, and tofu to support muscle function and repair.

5. **Nuts and Seeds:** Almonds, walnuts, and flaxseeds are rich in healthy fats and nutrients that can be beneficial for those with MS.

6. **Low-Fat Dairy (or Alternatives):** Opt for low-fat dairy products like yogurt or explore dairy-free alternatives like almond milk if lactose intolerance is a concern.

7. **Herbs and Spices:** Include herbs like turmeric, ginger, and rosemary for their anti-inflammatory properties and potential benefits for MS symptoms.

8. **Legumes:** Lentils, chickpeas, and beans are great sources of plant-based protein and fiber.

9. **Hydrating Foods:** Foods with high water content, such as watermelon and cucumbers, can help maintain hydration.

10. **Colorful Berries:** Berries like blueberries and strawberries are packed with antioxidants, which can combat inflammation.

11. **Herbal Teas:** Herbal teas, like green tea or chamomile, can offer soothing benefits and additional hydration.

## Foods to avoid

Just as there are foods that can be advantageous for managing multiple sclerosis, there are also items best kept in moderation or avoided entirely to support your well-being. Here are some foods to be cautious about:

1. **Processed Foods:** Highly processed foods often contain excessive levels of salt, unhealthy fats, and preservatives that can contribute to inflammation and energy fluctuations.

2. **Sugary Treats:** High-sugar foods and beverages can lead to blood sugar spikes and crashes, potentially exacerbating MS-related fatigue.

3. **Saturated Fats:** Foods high in saturated fats, like red meat and full-fat dairy, can promote inflammation and should be consumed in moderation.

4. **Trans Fats:** Trans fats, found in many fast food items and processed snacks, should be avoided due to their detrimental effects on the heart and overall health.

5. **Excessive Salt:** Excessive salt intake can lead to water retention and increased blood pressure. Reducing salt is essential for overall well-being.

6. **Gluten (if intolerant):** Some individuals with MS may have gluten sensitivities, which can

exacerbate symptoms. If intolerant, consider gluten-free options.

7. **Dairy (if lactose intolerant):** Lactose intolerance can be common in individuals with MS. If you're intolerant, choose lactose-free or dairy alternatives.

8. **Alcohol:** Excessive alcohol consumption can interact negatively with MS medications and may worsen symptoms. Moderate consumption is advisable.

9. **Caffeine (if sensitive):** While caffeine is generally safe, sensitive individuals may experience exacerbated MS symptoms like anxiety or sleep disturbances.

10. **Highly Spiced Foods:** Very spicy foods can sometimes trigger gastrointestinal issues, so it's essential to monitor your tolerance.

# Shopping List for Multiple Sclerosis Diet

## Fruits and Vegetables

- Fruits: Apples, bananas, berries, citrus fruits, grapes, melons, peaches, pears, plums
- Vegetables: Artichokes, asparagus, avocados, broccoli, Brussels sprouts, carrots, cauliflower, celery, cucumbers, eggplant, garlic, ginger, kale, leafy greens, mushrooms, onions, peppers, potatoes, spinach, squash, sweet potatoes, tomatoes, zucchini

## Grains

- Whole grains: Brown rice, whole-wheat pasta, quinoa, whole-wheat bread,
- Gluten-free options: Amaranth, buckwheat, millet, oats, quinoa, sorghum

## Legumes

- Beans: Black beans, chickpeas, kidney beans, lentils, pinto beans
- Legumes: Lentils, peas

## Nuts and Seeds

- Nuts: Almonds, cashews, hazelnuts, macadamia nuts, pecans, peanuts, pistachios, walnuts
- Seeds: Hemp seeds, pumpkin seeds, chia seeds, sesame seeds, sunflower seeds, flaxseeds

## Lean Protein Sources

- Fish: Fatty fish (salmon, tuna, mackerel), white fish (cod, flounder, tilapia)
- Poultry: Chicken, turkey
- Eggs: Free-range, omega-3 enriched
- Meat: Lean cuts of beef, lamb, pork
- Plant-based protein sources: Tofu, tempeh, lentils, beans, nuts, seeds

## Dairy and Dairy Alternatives

- Dairy: Milk, yogurt, cheese (choose low-fat or fat-free options)
- Dairy alternatives: Almond milk, soy milk, oat milk, rice milk

## Healthy Fats

- Olive oil: Extra virgin olive oil
- Avocado oil: Cold-pressed avocado oil
- Nut oils: Almond oil, walnut oil

## Herbs and Spices

- Fresh herbs: Basil, cilantro, parsley, rosemary, thyme
- Dried herbs: Oregano, paprika, sage, thyme
- Spices: Cinnamon, cumin, ginger, nutmeg, turmeric

## Other Healthy Ingredients

**Gluten-Free Flours for Baking:** Opt for gluten-free flour such as almond flour, coconut flour, rice flour, or a gluten-free flour blend. These options are suitable for people with gluten sensitivities.

- Honey or maple syrup: As natural sweeteners
- Fresh or frozen fruits and vegetables: For smoothies, snacks, and desserts

**Foods to Limit or Avoid**

- Red meat: Limit intake to 3 ounces per week
- Processed meats: Avoid hot dogs, sausages, bacon, lunch meats
- Full-fat dairy products: Choose fat-free or low-fat options
- Fried foods: Avoid fried foods or cook them using healthy oils
- Sugary drinks: Limit intake of soda, juice, and sweetened coffee or tea
- Processed snacks: Avoid chips, cookies, crackers, and other processed snacks
- Artificial sweeteners: Avoid aspartame, sucralose, and saccharin

# CHAPTER 2

## Breakfast Recipes for MS

## 1. Veggie Breakfast Burrito

**Preparation Time:** 20 minutes **Serves:** 2

**Ingredients:**

- 4 large eggs
- 1/4 cup diced bell peppers (any color)
- 1/4 cup diced onions
- 1/4 cup diced tomatoes
- 1/4 cup diced mushrooms
- 1/4 cup shredded cheddar cheese
- Salt and pepper to taste
- 2 whole-grain tortillas
- Salsa or hot sauce (optional)

**Nutritional Information:** Per serving: Calories: 330, Fat: 17g, Protein: 20g, Carbohydrates: 25g, Fiber: 3g

**Instructions:**

1. In a bowl, whisk the eggs and season with a pinch of salt and pepper.
2. In a non-stick skillet, heat a bit of oil over medium heat.
3. Add the diced bell peppers, onions, tomatoes, and mushrooms to the skillet. Stir-fry for about 5 minutes until the vegetables reach a tender state.
4. Pour the whisked eggs into the skillet with the sautéed veggies. Cook, with occasional stirring, until the eggs are set.
5. Distribute the shredded cheddar cheese on the eggs. Let it melt.
6. Warm the whole-grain tortillas in the skillet for a few seconds on each side.
7. Divide the scrambled egg mixture between the tortillas.
8. Optionally, add salsa or hot sauce for an extra kick.
9. Roll the tortillas, folding in the sides to make burritos.

**Serving Suggestions:** Serve the Veggie Breakfast Burritos with a side of fresh fruit, such as sliced melon or berries, for a balanced and satisfying morning meal.

## 2. Quinoa and Vegetable Breakfast Stir-Fry

**Preparation Time:** 25 minutes **Serves:** 2

**Ingredients:**

- 1/2 cup quinoa
- 1 cup water
- 2 tablespoons olive oil
- 1/4 cup diced bell peppers (any color)
- 1/4 cup diced onions
- 1/4 cup diced zucchini
- 1/4 cup diced cherry tomatoes
- 2 large eggs
- Salt and pepper to taste
- Fresh basil leaves for garnish (optional)

**Nutritional Information:** Per serving: Calories: 340, Fat: 15g, Protein: 12g, Carbohydrates: 38g, Fiber: 6g

**Instructions:**

1. Rinse the quinoa under cold water. Mix quinoa and water in a saucepan. Bring it to a boil, then lower the heat, cover, and let it simmer for roughly 15 minutes, or until the quinoa is done, and the water is fully absorbed.
2. Heat the olive oil over medium heat in a big skillet.
3. Add the diced bell peppers, onions, zucchini, and cherry tomatoes to the skillet. Sauté for about 5-7 minutes until the vegetables are tender.
4. Create space for the vegetables on one side of the skillet, and crack the eggs into the opposite side. Scramble the eggs until cooked.
5. Combine the cooked quinoa with the sautéed vegetables and scrambled eggs. Stir well to mix everything.
6. Season with salt and pepper to taste.

7.  Garnish with fresh basil leaves if desired.

**Serving Suggestions:** Serve the Quinoa and Vegetable Breakfast Stir-Fry with a side of Greek yogurt and a drizzle of honey for a wholesome and satisfying breakfast.

# 3. Chia Seed Pudding

**Preparation Time:** 10 minutes (plus chilling time)
**Serves:** 2

**Ingredients:**

- 1/4 cup chia seeds
- 1 cup unsweetened almond milk
- 1 tablespoon honey or maple syrup (adjust to taste)
- 1/2 teaspoon vanilla extract
- Fresh berries for topping (e.g., strawberries, blueberries, raspberries)
- Chopped nuts for garnish (e.g., almonds, walnuts)

**Nutritional Information:** Per serving: Calories: 180, Fat: 8g, Protein: 6g, Carbohydrates: 22g, Fiber: 9g

**Instructions:**

1. In a mixing bowl, combine the chia seeds, almond milk, honey (or maple syrup), and vanilla extract.
2. Whisk the ingredients together until well combined.
3. Seal the bowl and place it in the refrigerator for at least 4 hours or overnight, enabling the chia seeds to soak up the liquid and produce a pudding-style texture.
4. Before serving, stir the chia pudding to ensure it's evenly mixed.
5. Divide the pudding into serving dishes.
6. Top with fresh berries and chopped nuts.

**Serving Suggestions:** Chia Seed Pudding is a versatile breakfast option. You can customize it with your favorite toppings, such as sliced bananas, shredded coconut, or a drizzle of almond butter. Enjoy it as a nutritious and filling morning treat.

# 4. Banana and walnut pancakes

**Preparation Time:** 20 minutes **Serves:** 2

**Ingredients:**

- 1 ripe banana
- 2 large eggs
- 1/2 cup chopped walnuts
- 1/2 teaspoon vanilla extract
- 1/4 teaspoon ground cinnamon
- Cooking oil or butter for the skillet (if needed)

**Nutritional Information:** Per serving: Calories: 300, Fat: 22g, Protein: 10g, Carbohydrates: 21g, Fiber: 3g

**Instructions:**

1. Mash the ripe banana until it is smooth, in a mixing bowl.
2. Add the eggs, vanilla extract, and ground cinnamon to the mashed banana. Whisk until well combined.

3. Gently fold in the chopped walnuts.

4. Heat a non-stick skillet over medium heat. If needed, lightly grease the skillet with cooking oil or butter.

5. Pour a portion of the pancake batter into the skillet to create a pancake. Cook for approximately 2-3 minutes per side or until both sides are golden brown.

6. Make more pancakes by repeating the process with the remaining batter.

7. Serve the Banana and Walnut Pancakes with fresh fruit or a drizzle of honey if desired.

**Serving Suggestions:** These pancakes are delightful with a side of mixed berries, Greek yogurt, or a sprinkle of extra chopped walnuts. Enjoy them as a nutritious and satisfying breakfast option.

# 5. Scrambled tofu with spinach and cheese

**Preparation Time:** 15 minutes **Serves:** 2

**Ingredients:**

- 1 block (14 oz) firm tofu, crumbled
- 1 cup fresh spinach leaves
- 1/4 cup shredded cheddar cheese
- 1/4 teaspoon turmeric powder
- 1/4 teaspoon paprika
- Salt and pepper to taste
- Cooking oil or butter for the skillet (if needed)

**Nutritional Information:** Per serving: Calories: 220, Fat: 15g, Protein: 18g, Carbohydrates: 4g, Fiber: 1g

**Instructions:**

1. Heat a non-stick skillet over medium heat. If needed, lightly grease the skillet with cooking oil or butter.

2. Add the crumbled tofu to the skillet. Cook for about 5 minutes, stirring occasionally, until it starts to brown.

3. Sprinkle the turmeric, paprika, salt, and pepper over the tofu. Stir to evenly distribute the spices.

4. Add the fresh spinach leaves to the skillet and continue cooking for another 2-3 minutes or until the spinach wilts.

5. Sprinkle the shredded cheddar cheese over the tofu and spinach mixture. Cook for an additional 1-2 minutes until the cheese is fully melted.

6. Serve the Scrambled Tofu with Spinach and Cheese with whole-grain toast or tortillas, if desired.

**Serving Suggestions:** This tofu scramble pairs well with whole-grain toast, a side of sliced avocado, or a small fruit salad for a well-rounded and satisfying breakfast.

# 6. Smoked Salmon and Cucumber Wrap

**Preparation Time:** 10 minutes **Serves:** 2

**Ingredients:**

- 4 oz smoked salmon
- 1 small cucumber, thinly sliced
- 4 large lettuce leaves (e.g., butter or romaine lettuce)
- 2 tablespoons Greek yogurt
- 1 teaspoon fresh dill, chopped
- 1 teaspoon capers
- 1/2 lemon, sliced for garnish

**Nutritional Information:** Per serving: Calories: 150, Fat: 4g, Protein: 18g, Carbohydrates: 6g, Fiber: 1g

**Instructions:**

1. In a small bowl, combine the Greek yogurt and fresh dill to create a dill yogurt spread.
2. Lay out the large lettuce leaves, and spread a thin layer of the dill yogurt mixture on each leaf.

3. Place the thinly sliced cucumber on top of the yogurt spread.

4. Lay smoked salmon over the cucumber.

5. Sprinkle capers over the salmon.

6. Fold the lettuce leaves to make wraps.

7. Serve the Smoked Salmon and Cucumber Wraps with lemon slices for garnish.

**Serving Suggestions:** Pair these wraps with a side of fresh fruit or a simple green salad to create a light and satisfying breakfast or brunch option.

# 7. Buckwheat Pancakes

**Preparation Time:** 20 minutes **Serves:** 2

**Ingredients:**

- 1 cup buckwheat flour
- 1 teaspoon baking powder
- 1/4 teaspoon salt
- 1 tablespoon honey or maple syrup (adjust to taste)
- 1 cup unsweetened almond milk

- 1 large egg
- Cooking oil or butter for the skillet (if needed)

**Nutritional Information:** Per serving: Calories: 320, Fat: 6g, Protein: 11g, Carbohydrates: 60g, Fiber: 9g

**Instructions:**

1. In a mixing bowl, combine the buckwheat flour, baking powder, and salt.
2. In a separate bowl, whisk together the honey (or maple syrup), almond milk, and egg.
3. Mix the wet ingredients with the dry ingredients, and ensure they are well combined. The batter will be slightly lumpy.
4. Heat a non-stick skillet over medium heat. If needed, lightly grease the skillet with cooking oil or butter.
5. Pour a portion of the pancake batter into the skillet to create a pancake. Cook for approximately 2-3 minutes per side or until both sides are golden brown.
6. Make more pancakes by repeating the process with the remaining batter.

**Serving Suggestions:** Serve the Buckwheat Pancakes with a topping of fresh berries, a dollop of Greek yogurt, or a drizzle of honey for a hearty and nutritious breakfast.

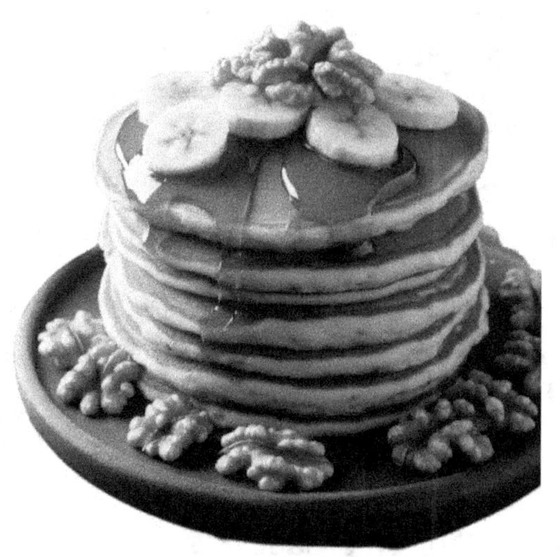

# CHAPTER 3

## Lunch Recipes for MS

## 1. Chicken Breast with Lentil Soup

**Preparation Time:** 30 minutes **Serves:** 2

**Ingredients:**

- 2 boneless, skinless chicken breasts
- 1 cup dried green or brown lentils
- 4 cups low-sodium chicken or vegetable broth
- 1 small onion, diced
- 2 carrots, diced
- 2 celery stalks, diced
- 2 cloves garlic, minced
- 1 teaspoon dried thyme
- Salt and pepper to taste
- Olive oil for cooking

**Nutritional Information:** Per serving: Calories: 320, Fat: 3g, Protein: 40g, Carbohydrates: 32g, Fiber: 12g

**Instructions:**

1. In a large pot, heat a bit of olive oil over medium heat.
2. Add the diced onions, celery, and carrots to the pot. For 5 minutes, stir-fry the vegetables until they start to become soft.
3. Add the minced garlic and dried thyme. Sauté for another minute, until the aroma is released.
4. Rinse the lentils and add them to the pot, along with the low-sodium broth. Bring to a boil.
5. Reduce the heat and let the lentil soup simmer for about 20-25 minutes or until the lentils are tender.
6. Season with salt and pepper to taste.
7. While the soup simmers, season the chicken breasts with salt and pepper.
8. Heat a separate skillet over medium-high heat and cook the chicken breasts for about 6-7 minutes on each side, or until they are cooked through.
9. Once the lentil soup is ready, serve it alongside the cooked chicken breasts.

**Serving Suggestions:** Serve the Chicken Breast with Lentil Soup with a side of steamed greens or a crisp green salad for a hearty and satisfying lunch.

## 2. Turkey and Avocado Sandwich on Gluten-free Bread

**Preparation Time:** 10 minutes **Serves:** 2

**Ingredients:**

- 4 slices of almond-flour bread (gluten-free)
- 6 oz turkey breast slices
- 1 ripe avocado, thinly sliced
- 1 small tomato, thinly sliced
- Lettuce leaves (e.g., butter or romaine)
- Dijon mustard or mayonnaise (optional)

**Nutritional Information:** Per serving: Calories: 280, Fat: 12g, Protein: 22g, Carbohydrates: 22g, Fiber: 8g

**Instructions:**

1. If desired, lightly toast the almond-flour bread slices.
2. Layer the turkey breast slices, avocado, tomato, and lettuce on two slices of bread.

3. Add Dijon mustard or mayonnaise, if desired.

4. Top each sandwich with the remaining slices of almond-flour bread.

5. Cut the sandwiches in half if preferred.

**Serving Suggestions:** Serve the Turkey and Avocado Sandwiches with a side of carrot sticks, cherry tomatoes, or a small fruit salad for a quick and satisfying lunch.

# 3. Cauliflower and Chickpea Curry

- **Preparation Time:** 20 minutes
- **Serves:** 4
- **Ingredients:**
    1. 1 head of cauliflower, cut into florets
    2. 1 can of chickpeas, drained and rinsed
    3. 1 onion, finely chopped
    4. 2 cloves of garlic, minced
    5. 1 can of diced tomatoes
    6. 1 can of coconut milk
    7. 2 tablespoons curry powder
    8. 1 teaspoon turmeric
    9. 1 teaspoon cumin

10. 1/2 teaspoon ginger

11. Salt and pepper to taste

12. Fresh cilantro for garnish

13. Cooked rice for serving

- **Nutritional Information (per serving):** Calories: 280, Protein: 9g, Carbohydrates: 34g, Fat: 12g, Fiber: 8g

- **Instructions:**

  1. In a large, deep skillet or a pot, heat some oil over medium heat.

  2. Add the chopped onion and garlic. Sauté until they appear transparent and their aroma is released.

  3. Stir in the cumin, curry powder, ginger, and turmeric Cook for an extra minute to release their aroma.

  4. Add the cauliflower florets and chickpeas to the pot, coating them with the spices and onions.

  5. Pour in the can of diced tomatoes and coconut milk. Stir well to combine all the ingredients.

6. Season with salt and pepper to taste. Reduce the heat to a simmer, cover, and cook for about 15 minutes or until the cauliflower is tender.

7. Taste and adjust the seasonings if necessary.

8. Serve the cauliflower and chickpea curry hot over cooked rice, garnished with fresh cilantro.

**Serving Suggestion:** Enjoy this flavorful and nutritious Cauliflower and Chickpea Curry as a delicious lunch option. It pairs wonderfully with a side of basmati rice or naan bread for a complete and satisfying meal.

# 4. Rice and Bean Burrito

**Preparation Time:** 20 minutes **Serves:** 2

**Ingredients:**

- 1 cup cooked brown rice
- 1 cup of drained and rinsed canned black beans

- 1/2 cup diced tomatoes
- 1/4 cup diced onions
- 1/4 cup diced bell peppers (any color)
- 1 teaspoon chili powder
- Salt and pepper to taste
- 2 whole-grain tortillas

**Nutritional Information:** Per serving: Calories: 320, Fat: 2g, Protein: 12g, Carbohydrates: 66g, Fiber: 10g

**Instructions:**

1. In a skillet, heat a bit of oil over medium heat.
2. Add the diced onions and bell peppers. Sauté for about 5 minutes until they start to soften.
3. Add the diced tomatoes and cook for an extra 2-3 minutes, stirring.
4. Add the cooked brown rice, black beans, chili powder, salt, and pepper to the skillet. Mix thoroughly and continue cooking until everything is all heated through.
5. Warm the whole-grain tortillas in the skillet for a few seconds on each side.

6. Divide the rice and bean mixture between the
   tortillas.

7. Roll up the tortillas to create burritos.

**Serving Suggestions:** Serve the Rice and Bean Burritos with a side of mixed greens, a dollop of Greek yogurt, or a salsa for a balanced and satisfying lunch.

# 5. Tuna and White Bean Salad

**Preparation Time:** 15 minutes **Serves:** 2

**Ingredients:**

- 1 can (6 oz) of tuna in water, drained and flaked
- 1 can (15 oz) of white beans (cannellini or navy beans), drained and rinsed
- 1/2 red onion, finely chopped
- 1 celery stalk, diced
- 1/4 cup chopped fresh parsley
- 2 tablespoons olive oil
- 2 tablespoons lemon juice
- Salt and pepper to taste

**Nutritional Information:** Per serving: Calories: 300, Fat: 10g, Protein: 25g, Carbohydrates: 28g, Fiber: 8g

**Instructions:**

1. In a large mixing bowl, combine the flaked tuna, white beans, chopped red onion, diced celery, and chopped fresh parsley.
2. Drizzle olive oil and lemon juice over the ingredients.
3. Gently toss everything together until well mixed.
4. Season with salt and pepper to taste.
5. Refrigerate for approximately 30 minutes before serving to allow the flavors to meld.

**Serving Suggestions:** It pairs well with whole-grain crackers, pita bread, or a side of fresh, crisp vegetables like cucumber and bell peppers.

# 6.  Mediterranean  Hummus  and Veggie Wrap

**Preparation Time:** 15 minutes **Serves:** 2

**Ingredients:**

- 2 whole-grain tortillas
- 1/2 cup hummus
- 1 cup diced cucumbers
- 1 cup diced tomatoes
- 1/4 cup diced red onions
- 1/4 cup sliced Kalamata olives
- 1/4 cup crumbled feta cheese
- Fresh mint leaves for garnish (optional)

**Nutritional Information:** Per serving: Calories: 320, Fat: 15g, Protein: 10g, Carbohydrates: 40g, Fiber: 8g

**Instructions:**

1. Lay out the whole-grain tortillas.
2. Spread a generous layer of hummus over each tortilla.

3. Divide the diced cucumbers, tomatoes, red onions, Kalamata olives, and crumbled feta cheese between the tortillas.

4. Optionally, garnish with fresh mint leaves.

5. Roll up the tortillas to create wraps.

**Serving Suggestions:** Serve with a side of sliced carrots, or whole cherry tomatoes for a quick and satisfying lunch.

# 7. Spinach and Goat Cheese Stuffed Chicken Breast

**Preparation Time:** 40 minutes **Serves:** 2

**Ingredients:**

- 2 boneless, skinless chicken breasts
- 2 cups fresh spinach leaves
- 1/4 cup crumbled goat cheese
- 1/4 cup diced sun-dried tomatoes
- 2 cloves garlic, minced
- 1/2 teaspoon dried oregano
- Salt and pepper to taste
- Cooking oil for searing

**Nutritional Information:** Per serving: Calories: 350, Fat: 15g, Protein: 40g, Carbohydrates: 6g, Fiber: 2g

**Instructions:**

1. Preheat the oven to 375°F (190°C).
2. In a mixing bowl, combine the fresh spinach leaves, crumbled goat cheese, diced sun-dried tomatoes, minced garlic, dried oregano, salt, and pepper.
3. Carefully cut an opening in every chicken breast to make a pocket.
4. Stuff the spinach and goat cheese mixture into the pockets of the chicken breasts.
5. Season the chicken breasts on the outside with additional salt and pepper.
6. Heat an oven-safe skillet over medium-high heat and add a bit of cooking oil.
7. Sear the stuffed chicken breasts for about 2-3 minutes on each side or until they are lightly browned.

8. Transfer the skillet to the preheated oven and bake for about 20-25 minutes until the chicken is cooked through and no longer pink inside.

**Serving Suggestions:** Serve the Spinach and Goat Cheese Stuffed Chicken Breasts with a side of quinoa, brown rice, or a green vegetable like steamed broccoli for a wholesome and satisfying lunch.

# CHAPTER 4

## Dinner Recipes for MS

## 1. Sesame Sockeye Salmon and Noodles

**Preparation Time:** 25 minutes **Serves:** 2

**Ingredients:**

- 2 sockeye salmon fillets
- 8 oz soba noodles
- 2 tablespoons sesame oil
- 2 tablespoons low-sodium soy sauce
- 1 tablespoon honey
- 1 clove garlic, minced
- 1/2 teaspoon grated ginger
- 1/2 teaspoon sesame seeds
- Sliced green onions for garnish

**Nutritional Information:** Per serving: Calories: 450, Fat: 15g, Protein: 30g, Carbohydrates: 45g, Fiber: 2g

**Instructions:**

1. Cook the soba noodles according to package instructions. Drain and set aside.
2. In a small bowl, whisk together sesame oil, low-sodium soy sauce, honey, minced garlic, grated ginger, and sesame seeds.
3. Season the sockeye salmon fillets with salt and pepper.
4. Heat a skillet on medium-high heat and include a small amount of oil.
5. Sear the salmon fillets for about 4-5 minutes on each side or until they are cooked to your liking. Brush with the sesame sauce during the last few minutes of cooking.
6. Toss the cooked soba noodles with the remaining sesame sauce.
7. Serve the salmon fillets on a bed of sesame noodles.
8. Garnish with sliced green onions.

**Serving Suggestions:** Pair the Sesame Sockeye Salmon and Noodles with a side of steamed broccoli, bok choy, or snap peas for a delicious and balanced dinner.

## 2. Ratatouille

**Preparation Time:** 45 minutes **Serves:** 4

**Ingredients:**

- 1 eggplant, diced
- 1 zucchini, diced
- 1 yellow bell pepper, diced
- 1 red bell pepper, diced
- 1 onion, finely chopped
- 2 cloves garlic, minced
- 2 cups diced tomatoes (canned or fresh)
- 2 tablespoons olive oil
- 1 teaspoon dried thyme
- 1 teaspoon dried oregano
- Salt and pepper to taste
- Fresh basil leaves for garnish (optional)

**Nutritional Information:** Per serving: Calories: 160, Fat: 6g, Protein: 3g, Carbohydrates: 26g, Fiber: 8g

**Instructions:**

1. Heat the olive oil over medium heat, in a big skillet.

2. Add the finely chopped onion and minced garlic. Keep sautéing for about 3 minutes until the onion appears translucent.

3. Add your diced eggplant, bell peppers, and zucchini to the skillet. Sauté for up to 5 minutes until your vegetables begin to soften.

4. Stir in your diced tomatoes, dried oregano, dried thyme, salt, and pepper. Mix well.

5. Cover the skillet and let the Ratatouille simmer for about 20-25 minutes, stirring occasionally, until the vegetables are tender.

6. If you prefer, you can opt to garnish with fresh basil leaves before serving.

**Serving Suggestions:** Ratatouille can be served as a side dish alongside grilled chicken, fish, or as a main course. It's versatile and pairs well with crusty bread or a side of cooked quinoa or couscous.

# 3. Eggplant Parmesan

**Preparation Time:** 60 minutes **Serves:** 4

**Ingredients:**

- 2 large eggplants, sliced into rounds
- 2 cups marinara sauce
- 2 cups shredded mozzarella cheese
- 1/2 cup grated Parmesan cheese
- 1 cup breadcrumbs (gluten-free if preferred)
- 2 eggs, beaten
- 1/4 cup fresh basil leaves
- Salt and pepper to taste
- Cooking oil for frying

**Nutritional Information:** Per serving: Calories: 450, Fat: 20g, Protein: 20g, Carbohydrates: 40g, Fiber: 7g

**Instructions:**

1. Preheat the oven to 375°F (190°C).
2. Dip each eggplant slice into the beaten eggs and then coat them with breadcrumbs.
3. Heat cooking oil in a skillet over medium-high heat and fry the eggplant slices for about 2-3

minutes on each side, or until they are golden brown. Lay them on paper towels to get rid of extra oil.

4.  Line a baking dish with a thin layer of marinara sauce.
5.  Arrange fried eggplant slices to form a layer over the sauce.
6.  Sprinkle a portion of mozzarella and Parmesan cheese over the eggplant.
7.  Add some fresh basil leaves, salt, and pepper.
8.  Repeat these layers until all the eggplant slices are used up.
9.  Finish with a layer of sauce and a generous topping of cheese.
10. Bake in the preheated oven for about 25-30 minutes until the cheese is bubbly and golden.

**Serving Suggestions:** Serve Eggplant Parmesan as a comforting and hearty dinner. It's great with a side of spaghetti or a green salad.

# 4. Mediterranean Baked Halibut

**Preparation Time:** 30 minutes **Serves:** 2

**Ingredients:**

- 2 halibut fillets
- 1 cup diced tomatoes (canned or fresh)
- 1/4 cup Kalamata olives, pitted and chopped
- 2 cloves garlic, minced
- 2 tablespoons olive oil
- 1/2 teaspoon dried oregano
- 1/2 teaspoon dried basil
- 1/4 teaspoon red pepper flakes (adjust to taste)
- Salt and pepper to taste
- Fresh parsley for garnish (optional)

**Nutritional Information:** Per serving: Calories: 280, Fat: 12g, Protein: 35g, Carbohydrates: 10g, Fiber: 3g

**Instructions:**

1. Preheat the oven to 375°F (190°C).
2. In a baking dish, combine the diced tomatoes, chopped Kalamata olives, minced garlic, olive

oil, dried oregano, dried basil, red pepper flakes, salt, and pepper.

3. Place the halibut fillets on top of the tomato mixture.

4. Drizzle a bit of olive oil over the halibut and season with additional salt and pepper.

5. Bake in the preheated oven for about 20-25 minutes until the halibut is cooked through and flakes easily.

6. Optionally, garnish with fresh parsley before serving.

**Serving Suggestions:** Mediterranean Baked Halibut pairs beautifully with a side of quinoa, couscous, or roasted vegetables. It's a flavorful and healthy dinner option.

## 5. Mushroom Risotto

**Preparation Time:** 45 minutes **Serves:** 4

**Ingredients:**

- 1 1/2 cups Arborio rice
- 8 oz cremini mushrooms, sliced

- 1 small onion, finely chopped
- 2 cloves garlic, minced
- 4 cups low-sodium vegetable broth
- 1/2 cup dry white wine (optional)
- 1/4 cup grated Parmesan cheese
- 2 tablespoons unsalted butter
- 2 tablespoons olive oil
- Fresh parsley for garnish
- Salt and pepper to taste

**Nutritional Information:** Per serving: Calories: 350, Fat: 8g, Protein: 7g, Carbohydrates: 60g, Fiber: 2g

**Instructions:**

1. In a big enough skillet, heat your olive oil and butter over medium heat.
2. Add the finely chopped onion and sauté for about 3 minutes until it becomes translucent.
3. Stir in the sliced cremini mushrooms and minced garlic. Cook for about 5 minutes until the mushrooms are tender.

4.  Add Arborio rice to the skillet and stir to coat it with the oil and butter. Cook for an additional 2-3 minutes.

5.  Optionally, pour in the white wine and cook until it's mostly absorbed.

6.  Begin adding the vegetable broth, one ladle at a time, stirring until the liquid is absorbed before adding more.

7.  Continue this process until the risotto is creamy and the rice is tender (about 20-25 minutes).

8.  Add the Parmesan cheese and sprinkle with salt and pepper to taste.

9.  Garnish with fresh parsley.

**Serving Suggestions:** Serve Mushroom Risotto as a delightful and filling dinner. Pair it with a green salad or steamed asparagus for a balanced meal.

# 6. Sweet Potato and Black Bean Tacos

**Preparation Time:** 30 minutes **Serves:** 2

**Ingredients:**

- 2 medium sweet potatoes, peeled and diced
- 1 can (15 oz) of drained and rinsed black beans.
- 1 red bell pepper, diced
- 1/2 red onion, finely chopped
- 2 cloves garlic, minced
- 1 teaspoon ground cumin
- 1/2 teaspoon chili powder (adjust to taste)
- Salt and pepper to taste
- 4 whole-grain tortillas
- Avocado slices and fresh cilantro for garnish (optional)

**Nutritional Information:** Per serving: Calories: 350, Fat: 2g, Protein: 10g, Carbohydrates: 70g, Fiber: 12g

**Instructions:**

1. In your big skillet, heat a touch of oil over medium heat.

2. Add the finely chopped red onion and sauté for about 3 minutes until it becomes translucent.

3. Stir in the ground cumin, minced garlic, and chili powder. Cook for an extra minute until fragrant.

4. Add the diced sweet potatoes to the skillet and sauté for about 10 minutes until they are tender.

5. Stir in the diced red bell pepper and black beans. Cook for an additional 5 minutes.

6. Season with salt and pepper to taste.

7. Warm the whole-grain tortillas in the skillet for a few seconds on each side.

8. Divide the sweet potato and black bean mixture between the tortillas.

9. Optionally, garnish with avocado slices and fresh cilantro.

**Serving Suggestions:** Serve the Sweet Potato and Black Bean Tacos with a side of Mexican rice or a fresh salsa for a satisfying and plant-based dinner.

# 7. Spaghetti Squash with Tomato Sauce

**Preparation Time:** 45 minutes **Serves:** 2

**Ingredients:**

- 1 medium spaghetti squash
- 2 cups tomato sauce (canned or homemade)
- 1/2 cup grated Parmesan cheese
- 2 cloves garlic, minced
- 1/2 teaspoon dried basil
- 1/2 teaspoon dried oregano
- Salt and pepper to taste
- Fresh basil leaves for garnish (optional)

**Nutritional Information:** Per serving: Calories: 280, Fat: 7g, Protein: 8g, Carbohydrates: 48g, Fiber: 8g

**Instructions:**

1. Preheat the oven to 375°F (190°C).
2. Cut the spaghetti squash in half lengthwise and remove the seeds.

3. Arrange the squash halves, with the cut side down, on a baking sheet. Roast in the preheated oven for about 30-35 minutes until the flesh is tender.

4. Use a fork to scrape the spaghetti-like strands from the squash and place them in a bowl.

5. In a separate saucepan, heat the tomato sauce and add the minced garlic, dried basil, dried oregano, salt, and pepper.

6. Simmer the sauce for about 10 minutes until it's heated through and flavorful.

7. Pour the tomato sauce over the spaghetti squash.

8. Sprinkle grated Parmesan cheese and fresh basil leaves as a garnish.

**Serving Suggestions:** Serve Spaghetti Squash with Tomato Sauce as a low-carb and nutritious dinner option. It's excellent on its own or paired with a side of mixed greens or a crisp cucumber salad.

# CHAPTER 5

# Desserts and Snacks for Multiple Sclerosis

## 1. Trail Mix Energy Bites

**Preparation Time:** 15 minutes **Makes:** Approximately 12 energy bites

**Ingredients:**

- 1 cup old-fashioned oats
- 1/2 cup of nut butter (e.g., almond, cashew, or peanut)
- 1/4 cup honey or maple syrup
- 1/2 cup dried fruits (e.g., cranberries, raisins, or apricots), finely chopped
- 1/4 cup mixed seeds (e.g., chia, flax, or sunflower seeds)
- 1/4 cup mini chocolate chips (optional)
- 1/2 teaspoon ground cinnamon
- 1/2 teaspoon vanilla extract
- A pinch of salt

**Nutritional Information:** Per energy bite (without chocolate chips): Calories: 100, Fat: 5g, Protein: 3g, Carbohydrates: 13g, Fiber: 2g

## Instructions:

1. In a large mixing bowl, combine the old-fashioned oats, nut butter, honey, or maple syrup, finely chopped dried fruits, mixed seeds, mini chocolate chips (if using), ground cinnamon, vanilla extract, and a pinch of salt.
2. Mix the ingredients until well combined.
3. Refrigerate the mixture for around 20-30 minutes so it becomes easier to handle.
4. Once it's chilled, scoop it into small portions and roll them into bite-sized balls.
5. Place the energy bites on a tray lined with parchment paper.
6. Refrigerate them for an additional 20-30 minutes until they firm up.
7. Store the Trail Mix Energy Bites in an airtight container in the refrigerator.

**Serving Suggestions:** Enjoy Trail Mix Energy Bites as a healthy snack to fuel your day. They are perfect for on-the-go energy and can be customized with your favorite ingredients.

## 2. Baked Apples with Cinnamon

**Preparation Time:** 45 minutes **Serves:** 4

**Ingredients:**

- 4 apples (e.g., Granny Smith or Honeycrisp)
- 1/4 cup chopped nuts (e.g., walnuts or almonds)
- 1/4 cup dried cranberries or raisins
- 1 teaspoon ground cinnamon
- 1/4 teaspoon nutmeg (optional)
- 2 tablespoons honey or maple syrup
- 1 tablespoon butter or coconut oil

**Nutritional Information:** Per serving (1 baked apple): Calories: 160, Fat: 5g, Protein: 2g, Carbohydrates: 30g, Fiber: 4g

**Instructions:**

1.  Preheat the oven to 350°F (175°C).

2.  Wash the apples, and then core them, leaving the bottom intact to create a well.

3.  In a mixing bowl, combine the chopped nuts, dried cranberries or raisins, ground cinnamon, and nutmeg (if using).

4.  Stuff each apple with the nut and dried fruit mixture.

5.  Drizzle honey or maple syrup over the stuffed apples.

6.  Place a small amount of butter or coconut oil on top of each apple.

7.  Arrange the apples in a baking dish, and add a bit of water to the dish to prevent sticking.

8.  Bake in the preheated oven for about 25-30 minutes or until the apples are tender.

**Serving Suggestions:** Serve Baked Apples with Cinnamon as a delightful and warm dessert. They can be enjoyed on their own or topped with a dollop of Greek yogurt or a sprinkle of granola for added texture and flavor.

# 3. Roasted Chickpeas

**Preparation Time:** 45 minutes **Serves:** 4

**Ingredients:**

- 2 cans (15 oz each) of chickpeas (garbanzo beans), drained and rinsed
- 2 tablespoons olive oil
- 1 teaspoon ground cumin
- 1 teaspoon paprika
- 1/2 teaspoon garlic powder
- Salt and pepper to taste

**Nutritional Information:** Per serving: Calories: 180, Fat: 7g, Protein: 8g, Carbohydrates: 20g, Fiber: 5g

**Instructions:**

1. Preheat the oven to 400°F (200°C).
2. Rinse and drain the chickpeas, and then pat them dry with a clean kitchen towel.
3. In a mixing bowl, toss the chickpeas with olive oil, ground cumin, paprika, garlic powder, salt, and pepper.

4.  Place the seasoned chickpeas on a baking sheet, in a single layer.

5.  Roast in the preheated oven for about 30-35 minutes, stirring them every 10 minutes, until they are crispy and golden.

6.  Let your roasted chickpeas cool before serving.

**Serving Suggestions:** Roasted Chickpeas make a satisfying and crunchy snack. They can be seasoned with various spices to suit your taste, and they are perfect for on-the-go or as a salad topper.

# 4.  Dark Chocolate and Almond Clusters

**Preparation Time:** 20 minutes **Serves:** 8

**Ingredients:**

- 8 oz dark chocolate (70% cocoa or higher)
- 1 cup whole almonds, roasted
- 1/4 cup dried cherries or cranberries
- A pinch of sea salt

**Nutritional Information:** Per serving (2 clusters): Calories: 180, Fat: 12g, Protein: 4g, Carbohydrates: 16g, Fiber: 3g

**Instructions:**

1. Line a baking sheet with parchment paper.
2. In a heatproof bowl, melt the dark chocolate using a microwave or a double boiler. Stir until smooth.
3. Stir the roasted whole almonds and dried cherries or cranberries into the melted chocolate.
4. With a spoon, create small clusters of the mixture on the prepared baking sheet
5. Sprinkle a touch of sea salt over each cluster.
6. Let the clusters cool and solidify at room temperature or in the refrigerator.

**Serving Suggestions:** Enjoy Dark Chocolate and Almond Clusters as a sweet and satisfying dessert. They are perfect for chocolate lovers and can also be a lovely homemade gift.

# 5. Chia Seed Berry Pudding

**Preparation Time:** 5 minutes (plus chilling time)

**Serves:** 2

**Ingredients:**

- 1/4 cup chia seeds
- 1 cup of almond milk or any healthy milk of your choice
- 1/2 teaspoon vanilla extract
- 1 tablespoon honey or maple syrup (adjust to taste)
- 1 cup mixed berries (e.g., strawberries, blueberries, raspberries)

**Nutritional Information:** Per serving: Calories: 180, Fat: 8g, Protein: 5g, Carbohydrates: 24g, Fiber: 11g

**Instructions:**

1. In a mixing bowl, whisk together chia seeds, almond milk, vanilla extract, and honey or maple syrup.

2. Cover the bowl and refrigerate the mixture for at least 2 hours or overnight to allow the chia seeds to absorb the liquid and thicken.

3. Once your chia pudding has thickened, stir it thoroughly.

4. Layer the chia pudding and mixed berries in serving glasses or bowls.

5. Optionally, drizzle a bit more honey or maple syrup on top.

**Serving Suggestions:** Chia Seed Berry Pudding is a healthy and filling dessert or snack. It's rich in fiber and antioxidants from the berries and chia seeds, making it a great choice for a guilt-free indulgence.

## 6. Apple Slices with Peanut Butter and Raisins

**Preparation Time:** 10 minutes **Serves:** 2

**Ingredients:**

- 2 medium apples (e.g., Gala or Fuji), cored and sliced

- 4 tablespoons natural peanut butter (or any preferred nut or seed butter)
- 2 tablespoons raisins
- A pinch of cinnamon (optional)

**Nutritional Information:** Per serving: Calories: 280, Fat: 14g, Protein: 7g, Carbohydrates: 35g, Fiber: 7g

**Instructions:**

1. Core and slice the apples into wedges.
2. Spread a generous layer of peanut butter on each apple slice.
3. Sprinkle raisins over the peanut butter.
4. Optionally, dust a pinch of cinnamon for added flavor.

**Serving Suggestions:** Enjoy Apple Slices with Peanut Butter and Raisins as a quick and satisfying snack. The combination of sweet apples, creamy peanut butter, and chewy raisins makes it a classic and nutritious choice.

# CHAPTER 6

## Beverages and Smoothies for MS

## 1. Berry and Flax Smoothie

**Preparation Time:** 5 minutes **Serves:** 2

**Ingredients:**

- 1 cup mixed berries (e.g., strawberries, blueberries, raspberries)
- 1 banana
- 1 tablespoon ground flaxseed
- 1 cup almond milk or any healthy milk of your choice
- 1/2 cup Greek yogurt
- 1 tablespoon honey (adjust to taste)
- Ice cubes (optional)

**Nutritional Information:** Per serving: Calories: 200, Fat: 5g, Protein: 7g, Carbohydrates: 35g, Fiber: 7g

**Instructions:**

1. Place mixed berries, banana, ground flaxseed, almond milk, Greek yogurt, and honey in a blender.

2. Optionally, add ice cubes for a colder and thicker smoothie.

3. Blend until all ingredients are well combined and the smoothie is creamy.

4. Taste it and, if required, enhance the sweetness by adding more honey.

**Serving Suggestions:** Enjoy the Berry and Flax Smoothie as a refreshing and nutritious beverage. It's perfect for a quick breakfast or as a post-workout energy booster.

# 2. Homemade Vegetable Juice

**Preparation Time:** 10 minutes **Serves:** 2

**Ingredients:**

- 4 large carrots, peeled and chopped
- 2 stalks celery, chopped
- 2 cucumbers, peeled and chopped
- 2 large tomatoes, chopped
- 1 red bell pepper, chopped
- 1/2 lemon, juiced
- A touch of salt and black pepper (if you like).

**Nutritional Information:** Per serving: Calories: 80, Fat: 0.5g, Protein: 2g, Carbohydrates: 18g, Fiber: 5g

**Instructions:**

1. Place the chopped carrots, celery, cucumbers, tomatoes, and red bell pepper in a juicer.
2. Juice all the vegetables until you have a fresh and vibrant homemade vegetable juice.
3. Optionally, add a pinch of salt and black pepper for added flavor.
4. Squeeze the lemon juice into the vegetable juice and stir.

**Serving Suggestions:** It's best enjoyed fresh and can be served as a breakfast beverage or as a refreshing drink at any time of the day.

# 3. Turmeric Golden Milk

**Preparation Time:** 10 minutes **Serves:** 2

**Ingredients:**

- 2 cups of unsweetened almond milk (or any other healthy milk you like)
- 1 teaspoon ground turmeric

- 1/2 teaspoon ground cinnamon
- 1/4 teaspoon ground ginger
- A pinch of black pepper
- 1 tablespoon honey or maple syrup (adjust to taste)
- 1/2 teaspoon vanilla extract

**Nutritional Information:** Per serving: Calories: 80, Fat: 2g, Protein: 1g, Carbohydrates: 15g, Fiber: 2g

**Instructions:**

1. Place the unsweetened almond milk in a saucepan and heat it over medium heat. Add the ground turmeric, ground cinnamon, ground ginger, a pinch of black pepper, honey or maple syrup, and vanilla extract.
2. Whisk the ingredients together and heat until the mixture is hot but not boiling.
3. Remove from heat and strain to remove any undissolved spices.
4. Pour the Turmeric Golden Milk into mugs and serve warm.

**Serving Suggestions:**

Turmeric Golden Milk is a comforting and soothing beverage. It's often enjoyed in the evening as a warm and relaxing drink.

# 4. Iced Herbal Tea

**Preparation Time:** 15 minutes (including chilling time) **Serves:** 4

**Ingredients:**

- 4 herbal tea bags (e.g., chamomile, peppermint, or hibiscus)
- 4 cups boiling water
- 2 tablespoons honey (adjust to taste)
- Fresh lemon slices and mint leaves for garnish (optional)
- Ice cubes

**Nutritional Information:** Per serving: Calories: 15, Fat: 0g, Protein: 0g, Carbohydrates: 4g, Fiber: 0g

**Instructions:**

1. Put the herbal tea bags in a heat-resistant pitcher.
2. Pour 4 cups of boiling water over the tea bags.
3. Allow the tea to steep for about 5-7 minutes, or according to the tea's package instructions.
4. Remove the tea bags and discard them.
5. Stir in honey to sweeten the tea (adjust to your taste).
6. Allow the tea to cool to room temperature.
7. Refrigerate the tea until it's well chilled.
8. Serve the Iced Herbal Tea over ice cubes.
9. Optionally, garnish with fresh lemon slices and mint leaves.

**Serving Suggestions:**

Iced Herbal Tea is a refreshing and caffeine-free beverage. It's perfect for warm days or as a calming and soothing choice in the evening. Customize it with your favorite herbal tea flavors.

# 5. Kale and pineapple juice

**Preparation Time:** 10 minutes **Serves:** 2

**Ingredients:**

- 4 cups fresh kale leaves, stems removed
- 2 cups fresh pineapple chunks
- 1 cucumber, peeled and chopped
- 1 lime, peeled
- 1 green apple, cored and chopped
- A pinch of salt (optional)

**Nutritional Information:** Per serving: Calories: 100, Fat: 0.5g, Protein: 2g, Carbohydrates: 25g, Fiber: 4g

**Instructions:**

1. Prepare the ingredients by washing the kale leaves, peeling the cucumber and lime, and chopping the pineapple and green apple.
2. Place all the prepared ingredients in a juicer.
3. Optionally, add a pinch of salt for added flavor.
4. Juice all the ingredients until you have a vibrant and refreshing kale and pineapple juice.
5. Stir well and serve immediately.

**Serving Suggestions:**

Kale and Pineapple Juice is a nutrient-packed and green elixir. Enjoy it as a morning pick-me-up or as a hydrating beverage any time of the day.

# 6. Cranberry and apple cider

**Preparation Time:** 10 minutes **Serves:** 4

**Ingredients:**

- 2 cups unsweetened cranberry juice
- 2 cups apple cider
- 1/4 cup freshly squeezed orange juice
- 1/2 teaspoon ground cinnamon
- Orange slices for garnish (optional)
- Ice cubes

**Nutritional Information:** Per serving: Calories: 100, Fat: 0g, Protein: 0g, Carbohydrates: 25g, Fiber: 1g

**Instructions:**

1. In a pitcher, combine unsweetened cranberry juice, apple cider, freshly squeezed orange juice, and ground cinnamon.

2. Stir well to mix all the flavors.

3. Optionally, add ice cubes to chill the beverage.

4. Serve the Cranberry and Apple Cider in glasses.

5. Garnish with orange slices for a citrusy touch.

**Serving Suggestions:**

It's perfect for holiday gatherings or as a refreshing choice on a warm day. Adjust the sweetness by adding more or less orange juice to suit your taste.

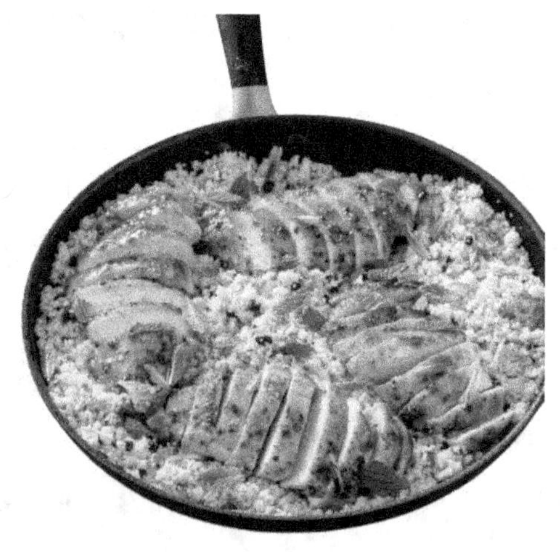

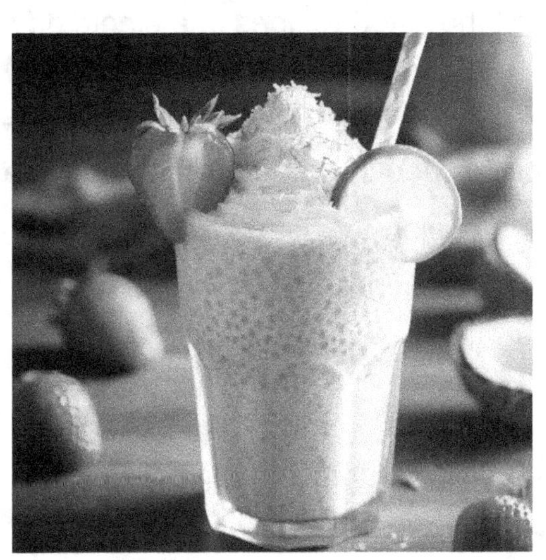

# CHAPTER 7

# 30 days Meal Plan

Please note that the provided meal plan is a sample and should not be interpreted as a recommendation to consume all the listed recipes in a single day.

The purpose of this meal plan is to offer inspiration and guidance for healthy meal preparation. Feel free to customize this plan further to suit your preferences and dietary requirements.

**Day 1:**

- **Breakfast:** Veggie Breakfast Burrito
- **Lunch:** Chicken Breast with Lentil Soup
- **Dinner:** Sesame Sockeye Salmon and Noodles
- **Dessert:** Trail Mix Energy Bites
- **Drink:** Berry and Flax Smoothie

**Day 2:**

- **Breakfast:** Chia Seed Berry Pudding
- **Lunch:** Turkey and Avocado Sandwich on Almond-Flour Bread
- **Dinner:** Ratatouille
- **Snack:** Roasted Chickpeas
- **Drink:** Homemade Vegetable Juice

**Day 3:**

- **Breakfast:** Buckwheat Pancakes
- **Lunch:** Quinoa Salad with Roasted Vegetables
- **Dinner:** Eggplant Parmesan
- **Dessert:** Dark Chocolate and Almond Clusters
- **Drink:** Turmeric Golden Milk

**Day 4:**

- **Breakfast:** Scrambled Tofu with Spinach and Cheese
- **Lunch:** Tuna and White Bean Salad

- **Dinner:** Mediterranean Baked Halibut
- **Snack:** Baked Apples with Cinnamon
- **Drink:** Iced Herbal Tea

**Day 5:**

- **Breakfast:** Quinoa and Vegetable Breakfast Stir-Fry
- **Lunch:** Spinach and Goat Cheese Stuffed Chicken Breast
- **Dinner:** Mushroom Risotto
- **Dessert:** Chia Seed Berry Pudding
- **Drink:** Kale and Pineapple Juice

**Day 6:**

- **Breakfast:** Veggie Breakfast Burrito
- **Lunch:** Chicken Breast with Lentil Soup
- **Dinner:** Sweet Potato and Black Bean Tacos
- **Snack:** Trail Mix Energy Bites
- **Drink:** Cranberry and Apple Cider

**Day 7:**

- **Breakfast:** Chia Seed Berry Pudding

- **Lunch:** Turkey and Avocado Sandwich on Almond-Flour Bread
- **Dinner:** Spaghetti Squash with Tomato Sauce
- **Dessert:** Dark Chocolate and Almond Clusters
- **Drink:** Berry and Flax Smoothie

**Day 8:**

- **Breakfast:** Buckwheat Pancakes
- **Lunch:** Quinoa Salad with Roasted Vegetables
- **Dinner:** Ratatouille
- **Snack:** Roasted Chickpeas
- **Drink:** Homemade Vegetable Juice

**Day 9:**

- **Breakfast:** Scrambled Tofu with Spinach and Cheese
- **Lunch:** Tuna and White Bean Salad
- **Dinner:** Mediterranean Baked Halibut
- **Dessert:** Baked Apples with Cinnamon
- **Drink:** Turmeric Golden Milk

**Day 10:**

- **Breakfast:** Quinoa and Vegetable Breakfast Stir-Fry
- **Lunch:** Spinach and Goat Cheese Stuffed Chicken Breast
- **Dinner:** Mushroom Risotto
- **Snack:** Trail Mix Energy Bites
- **Drink:** Iced Herbal Tea

**Day 11:**

- **Breakfast:** Veggie Breakfast Burrito
- **Lunch:** Chicken Breast with Lentil Soup
- **Dinner:** Sweet Potato and Black Bean Tacos
- **Dessert:** Chia Seed Berry Pudding
- **Drink:** Kale and Pineapple Juice

**Day 12:**

- **Breakfast:** Chia Seed Berry Pudding
- **Lunch:** Turkey and Avocado Sandwich on Almond-Flour Bread
- **Dinner:** Spaghetti Squash with Tomato Sauce
- **Snack:** Roasted Chickpeas
- **Drink:** Cranberry and Apple Cider

**Day 13:**

- **Breakfast:** Buckwheat Pancakes
- **Lunch:** Quinoa Salad with Roasted Vegetables
- **Dinner:** Ratatouille
- **Dessert:** Dark Chocolate and Almond Clusters
- **Drink:** Berry and Flax Smoothie

**Day 14:**

- **Breakfast:** Scrambled Tofu with Spinach and Cheese
- **Lunch:** Tuna and White Bean Salad
- **Dinner:** Mediterranean Baked Halibut
- **Snack:** Baked Apples with Cinnamon
- **Drink:** Homemade Vegetable Juice

**Day 15:**

- **Breakfast:** Quinoa and Vegetable Breakfast Stir-Fry
- **Lunch:** Spinach and Goat Cheese Stuffed Chicken Breast
- **Dinner:** Mushroom Risotto

- **Dessert:** Chia Seed Berry Pudding
- **Drink:** Turmeric Golden Milk

## Day 16:

- **Breakfast:** Veggie Breakfast Burrito
- **Lunch:** Chicken Breast with Lentil Soup
- **Dinner:** Sweet Potato and Black Bean Tacos
- **Snack:** Trail Mix Energy Bites
- **Drink:** Iced Herbal Tea

## Day 17:

- **Breakfast:** Chia Seed Berry Pudding
- **Lunch:** Turkey and Avocado Sandwich on Almond-Flour Bread
- **Dinner:** Spaghetti Squash with Tomato Sauce
- **Dessert:** Dark Chocolate and Almond Clusters
- **Drink:** Kale and Pineapple Juice

## Day 18:

- **Breakfast:** Buckwheat Pancakes
- **Lunch:** Quinoa Salad with Roasted Vegetables

- **Dinner:** Ratatouille
- **Snack:** Roasted Chickpeas
- **Drink:** Cranberry and Apple Cider

**Day 19:**

- **Breakfast:** Scrambled Tofu with Spinach and Cheese
- **Lunch:** Tuna and White Bean Salad
- **Dinner:** Mediterranean Baked Halibut
- **Dessert:** Baked Apples with Cinnamon
- **Drink:** Berry and Flax Smoothie

**Day 20:**

- **Breakfast:** Quinoa and Vegetable Breakfast Stir-Fry
- **Lunch:** Spinach and Goat Cheese Stuffed Chicken Breast
- **Dinner:** Mushroom Risotto
- **Snack:** Trail Mix Energy Bites
- **Drink:** Homemade Vegetable Juice

**Day 21:**

- **Breakfast:** Veggie Breakfast Burrito

- **Lunch:** Chicken Breast with Lentil Soup
- **Dinner:** Sweet Potato and Black Bean Tacos
- **Dessert:** Chia Seed Berry Pudding
- **Drink:** Turmeric Golden Milk

## Day 22:

- **Breakfast:** Chia Seed Berry Pudding
- **Lunch:** Turkey and Avocado Sandwich on Almond-Flour Bread
- **Dinner:** Spaghetti Squash with Tomato Sauce
- **Snack:** Roasted Chickpeas
- **Drink:** Berry and Flax Smoothie

## Day 23:

- **Breakfast:** Buckwheat Pancakes
- **Lunch:** Quinoa Salad with Roasted Vegetables
- **Dinner:** Ratatouille
- **Dessert:** Dark Chocolate and Almond Clusters
- **Drink:** Kale and Pineapple Juice

## Day 24:

- **Breakfast:** Scrambled Tofu with Spinach and Cheese
- **Lunch:** Tuna and White Bean Salad
- **Dinner:** Mushroom Risotto
- **Snack:** Roasted Chickpeas
- **Drink:** Cranberry and Apple Cider

**Day 25:**

- **Breakfast:** Quinoa and Vegetable Breakfast Stir-Fry
- **Lunch:** Spinach and Goat Cheese Stuffed Chicken Breast
- **Dinner:** Sweet Potato and Black Bean Tacos
- **Dessert:** Chia Seed Berry Pudding
- **Drink:** Turmeric Golden Milk

**Day 26:**

- **Breakfast:** Veggie Breakfast Burrito
- **Lunch:** Chicken Breast with Lentil Soup
- **Dinner:** Sesame Sockeye Salmon and Noodles
- **Snack:** Trail Mix Energy Bites

- **Drink:** Iced Herbal Tea

**Day 27:**

- **Breakfast:** Chia Seed Berry Pudding
- **Lunch:** Turkey and Avocado Sandwich on Almond-Flour Bread
- **Dinner:** Ratatouille
- **Dessert:** Dark Chocolate and Almond Clusters
- **Drink:** Homemade Vegetable Juice

**Day 28:**

- **Breakfast:** Buckwheat Pancakes
- **Lunch:** Quinoa Salad with Roasted Vegetables
- **Dinner:** Eggplant Parmesan
- **Snack:** Roasted Chickpeas
- **Drink:** Turmeric Golden Milk

**Day 29:**

- **Breakfast:** Scrambled Tofu with Spinach and Cheese
- **Lunch:** Tuna and White Bean Salad

- **Dinner:** Mediterranean Baked Halibut
- **Dessert:** Baked Apples with Cinnamon
- **Drink:** Iced Herbal Tea

**Day 30:**

- **Breakfast:** Quinoa and Vegetable Breakfast Stir-Fry
- **Lunch:** Spinach and Goat Cheese Stuffed Chicken Breast
- **Dinner:** Spaghetti Squash with Tomato Sauce
- **Snack:** Trail Mix Energy Bites
- **Drink:** Kale and Pineapple Juice

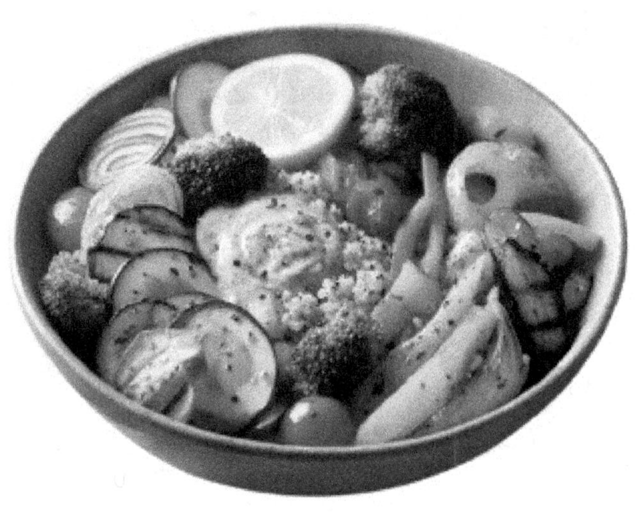

# CHAPTER 8

## Conclusion

In this cookbook, we've explored a world of culinary possibilities designed to support individuals living with multiple sclerosis. I understand the importance of making dietary choices that can help alleviate symptoms, improve energy levels, and enhance overall well-being.

**"Multiple Sclerosis Anti-Inflammatory Cookbook"** has been crafted with care to provide you with a wide range of delicious and nutritious recipes that align with the principles of a multiple sclerosis diet.

Our journey began with a deep dive into the principles of the multiple sclerosis diet, understanding the foods that can contribute to better health and those that are best avoided.

I also provided you with a comprehensive shopping list to ensure you have everything you need to embark on this dietary adventure.

Throughout the book, you've discovered a variety of breakfast, lunch, and dinner options that are not only flavorful but also designed to support your health. I've included delightful desserts and snacks, showing that living with multiple sclerosis doesn't mean sacrificing the joy of eating.

The beverage and smoothie recipes offer refreshing and hydrating options, providing a satisfying accompaniment to your meals or a pick-me-up during the day.

In closing, I hope this cookbook becomes a valuable resource in your journey to better health and well-being. My goal is to empower you to make mindful dietary choices while still savoring delicious meals.

I encourage you to explore these recipes, tailor them to your preferences, and embark on a path to a healthier and happier life.

Remember, the journey to better health is unique for each person, and it's essential to consult with your healthcare provider before making significant dietary changes.

As you navigate this path, may you find nourishment, joy, and the strength to face each day with a positive outlook and an empowered spirit.

Thank you for choosing the **"Multiple Sclerosis Anti-Inflammatory Cookbook."** We wish you good health and the joy of savoring every bite.